THIS BELONGS TO:

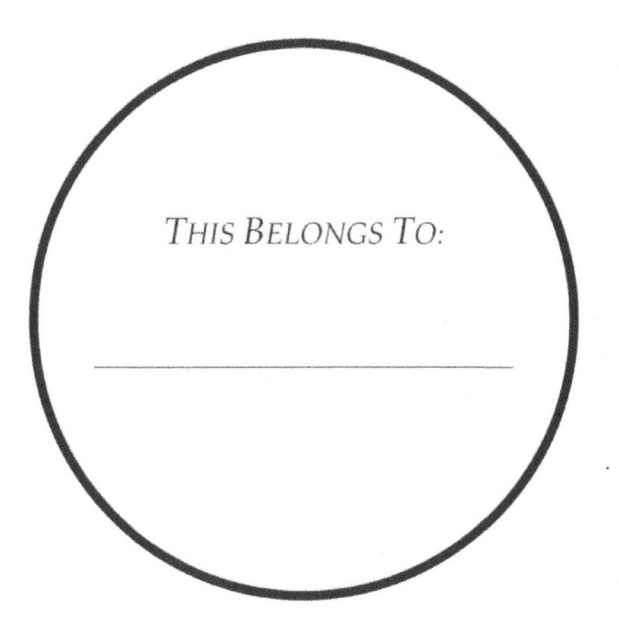

_____

Dog Health Record

Breed			Groomer		
Veterinarian		Emergency Veterinary Services			
Date	Physical Test Result	Fecal Test Result	Wormer Given	Heartworms Tests Results	Surgery

Important observations

Dog Health Record

Breed				Groomer		
Veterinarian			Emergency Veterinary Services			
Date	Physical Test Result	Fecal Test Result	Wormer Given	Heartworms Tests Results	Surgery	

Important observations

Dog Health Record

Breed				Groomer		
Veterinarian			Emergency Veterinary Services			
Date	Physical Test Result	Fecal Test Result	Wormer Given	Heartworms Tests Results	Surgery

Important observations

Dog Health Record

Breed				Groomer		
Veterinarian			Emergency Veterinary Services			
Date	Physical Test Result	Fecal Test Result	Wormer Given	Heartworms Tests Results	Surgery

Important observations

Dog Health Record

Breed			Groomer		
Veterinarian		Emergency Veterinary Services			
Date	Physical Test Result	Fecal Test Result	Wormer Given	Heartworms Tests Results	Surgery

Important observations

Dog Health Record

Breed				Groomer		
Veterinarian			Emergency Veterinary Services			
Date	Physical Test Result	Fecal Test Result	Wormer Given	Heartworms Tests Results	Surgery	

Important observations

Dog Health Record

Breed				Groomer	
Veterinarian		Emergency Veterinary Services			
Date	Physical Test Result	Fecal Test Result	Wormer Given	Heartworms Tests Results	Surgery

Important observations

Dog Health Record

Breed				Groomer		
Veterinarian			Emergency Veterinary Services			
Date	Physical Test Result	Fecal Test Result	Wormer Given	Heartworms Tests Results	Surgery	

Important observations

Dog Health Record

Breed				Groomer		
Veterinarian			Emergency Veterinary Services			
Date	Physical Test Result	Fecal Test Result	Wormer Given	Heartworms Tests Results	Surgery	

Important observations

Dog Health Record

Breed				Groomer	
Veterinarian			Emergency Veterinary Services		
Date	Physical Test Result	Fecal Test Result	Wormer Given	Heartworms Tests Results	Surgery

Important observations

Dog Health Record

Breed				Groomer	
Veterinarian		Emergency Veterinary Services			
Date	Physical Test Result	Fecal Test Result	Wormer Given	Heartworms Tests Results	Surgery

Important observations

Dog Health Record

Breed			Groomer		
Veterinarian		Emergency Veterinary Services			
Date	Physical Test Result	Fecal Test Result	Wormer Given	Heartworms Tests Results	Surgery

Important observations

Dog Health Record

Breed			Groomer		
Veterinarian		Emergency Veterinary Services			
Date	Physical Test Result	Fecal Test Result	Wormer Given	Heartworms Tests Results	Surgery

Important observations

Dog Health Record

Breed				Groomer		
Veterinarian			Emergency Veterinary Services			
Date	Physical Test Result	Fecal Test Result	Wormer Given	Heartworms Tests Results	Surgery	

Important observations

Dog Health Record

Breed				Groomer	
Veterinarian		Emergency Veterinary Services			
Date	Physical Test Result	Fecal Test Result	Wormer Given	Heartworms Tests Results	Surgery

Important observations

Dog Health Record

Breed			Groomer		
Veterinarian		Emergency Veterinary Services			
Date	Physical Test Result	Fecal Test Result	Wormer Given	Heartworms Tests Results	Surgery

Important observations

Dog Health Record

Breed				Groomer		
Veterinarian			Emergency Veterinary Services			
Date	Physical Test Result	Fecal Test Result	Wormer Given	Heartworms Tests Results	Surgery	

Important observations

Dog Health Record

Breed				Groomer	
Veterinarian			Emergency Veterinary Services		
Date	Physical Test Result	Fecal Test Result	Wormer Given	Heartworms Tests Results	Surgery

Important observations

Dog Health Record

Breed				Groomer		
Veterinarian			Emergency Veterinary Services			
Date	Physical Test Result	Fecal Test Result	Wormer Given	Heartworms Tests Results		Surgery

Important observations

Dog Health Record

Breed				Groomer		
Veterinarian			Emergency Veterinary Services			
Date	Physical Test Result	Fecal Test Result	Wormer Given	Heartworms Tests Results	Surgery	

Important observations

Dog Health Record

Breed				Groomer		
Veterinarian			Emergency Veterinary Services			
Date	Physical Test Result	Fecal Test Result	Wormer Given	Heartworms Tests Results	Surgery

Important observations

Dog Health Record

Breed		Groomer			
Veterinarian		Emergency Veterinary Services			
Date	Physical Test Result	Fecal Test Result	Wormer Given	Heartworms Tests Results	Surgery

Important observations

Dog Health Record

Breed			Groomer		
Veterinarian		Emergency Veterinary Services			
Date	Physical Test Result	Fecal Test Result	Wormer Given	Heartworms Tests Results	Surgery

Important observations

Dog Health Record

Breed			Groomer		
Veterinarian		Emergency Veterinary Services			
Date	Physical Test Result	Fecal Test Result	Wormer Given	Heartworms Tests Results	Surgery

Important observations

Dog Health Record

Breed			Groomer		
Veterinarian		Emergency Veterinary Services			
Date	Physical Test Result	Fecal Test Result	Wormer Given	Heartworms Tests Results	Surgery

Important observations

Dog Health Record

Breed			Groomer			
Veterinarian		Emergency Veterinary Services				
Date	Physical Test Result	Fecal Test Result	Wormer Given	Heartworms Tests Results	Surgery	

Important observations

Dog Health Record

Breed
Veterinarian
Groomer
Emergency Veterinary Services

Date	Physical Test Result	Fecal Test Result	Wormer Given	Heartworms Tests Results	Surgery

Important observations

Dog Health Record

Breed				Groomer	
Veterinarian		Emergency Veterinary Services			
Date	Physical Test Result	Fecal Test Result	Wormer Given	Heartworms Tests Results	Surgery

Important observations

Dog Health Record

Breed: _____ **Groomer:** _____

Veterinarian: _____ **Emergency Veterinary Services:** _____

Date	Physical Test Result	Fecal Test Result	Wormer Given	Heartworms Tests Results	Surgery

Important observations

Dog Health Record

Breed				Groomer		
Veterinarian			Emergency Veterinary Services			
Date	Physical Test Result	Fecal Test Result	Wormer Given	Heartworms Tests Results	Surgery

Important observations

Dog Health Record

Breed				Groomer		
Veterinarian			Emergency Veterinary Services			
Date	Physical Test Result	Fecal Test Result	Wormer Given	Heartworms Tests Results	Surgery	

Important observations

Dog Health Record

Breed				Groomer		
Veterinarian			Emergency Veterinary Services			
Date	Physical Test Result	Fecal Test Result	Wormer Given	Heartworms Tests Results	Surgery	

Important observations

Dog Health Record

Breed			Groomer	
Veterinarian		Emergency Veterinary Services		
Date	Physical Test Result	Fecal Test Result	Wormer Given	Heartworms Tests Results	Surgery

Important observations

Dog Health Record

Breed				Groomer		
Veterinarian			Emergency Veterinary Services			
Date	Physical Test Result	Fecal Test Result	Wormer Given	Heartworms Tests Results	Surgery

Important observations

Dog Health Record

Breed			Groomer		
Veterinarian		Emergency Veterinary Services			
Date	Physical Test Result	Fecal Test Result	Wormer Given	Heartworms Tests Results	Surgery

Important observations

Dog Health Record

Breed				Groomer		
Veterinarian			Emergency Veterinary Services			
Date	Physical Test Result	Fecal Test Result	Wormer Given	Heartworms Tests Results	Surgery

Important observations

Dog Health Record

Breed				Groomer		
Veterinarian			Emergency Veterinary Services			
Date	Physical Test Result	Fecal Test Result	Wormer Given	Heartworms Tests Results	Surgery	

Important observations

Dog Health Record

Breed				Groomer		
Veterinarian			Emergency Veterinary Services			
Date	Physical Test Result	Fecal Test Result	Wormer Given	Heartworms Tests Results	Surgery	

Important observations

Dog Health Record

Breed				Groomer		
Veterinarian			Emergency Veterinary Services			
Date	Physical Test Result	Fecal Test Result	Wormer Given	Heartworms Tests Results		Surgery

Important observations

Dog Health Record

Breed				Groomer		
Veterinarian			Emergency Veterinary Services			
Date	Physical Test Result	Fecal Test Result	Wormer Given	Heartworms Tests Results	Surgery

Important observations

Dog Health Record

Breed				Groomer		
Veterinarian			Emergency Veterinary Services			
Date	Physical Test Result	Fecal Test Result	Wormer Given	Heartworms Tests Results	Surgery	

Important observations

Dog Health Record

Breed			Groomer		
Veterinarian		Emergency Veterinary Services			
Date	Physical Test Result	Fecal Test Result	Wormer Given	Heartworms Tests Results	Surgery

Important observations

Dog Health Record

Breed				Groomer		
Veterinarian			Emergency Veterinary Services			
Date	Physical Test Result	Fecal Test Result	Wormer Given	Heartworms Tests Results	Surgery	

Important observations

Dog Health Record

Breed			Groomer		
Veterinarian		Emergency Veterinary Services			
Date	Physical Test Result	Fecal Test Result	Wormer Given	Heartworms Tests Results	Surgery

Important observations

Dog Health Record

Breed				Groomer		
Veterinarian			Emergency Veterinary Services			
Date	Physical Test Result	Fecal Test Result	Wormer Given	Heartworms Tests Results	Surgery

Important observations

Dog Health Record

Breed				Groomer		
Veterinarian			Emergency Veterinary Services			
Date	Physical Test Result	Fecal Test Result	Wormer Given	Heartworms Tests Results	Surgery	

Important observations

Dog Health Record

Breed				Groomer		
Veterinarian		Emergency Veterinary Services				
Date	Physical Test Result	Fecal Test Result	Wormer Given	Heartworms Tests Results	Surgery

Important observations

Dog Health Record

Breed				Groomer		
Veterinarian			Emergency Veterinary Services			
Date	Physical Test Result	Fecal Test Result	Wormer Given	Heartworms Tests Results		Surgery

Important observations

Dog Health Record

Breed				Groomer		
Veterinarian			Emergency Veterinary Services			
Date	Physical Test Result	Fecal Test Result	Wormer Given	Heartworms Tests Results	Surgery	

Important observations

Dog Health Record

Breed				Groomer		
Veterinarian			Emergency Veterinary Services			
Date	Physical Test Result	Fecal Test Result	Wormer Given	Heartworms Tests Results	Surgery	

Important observations

Dog Health Record

Breed				Groomer		
Veterinarian			Emergency Veterinary Services			
Date	Physical Test Result	Fecal Test Result	Wormer Given	Heartworms Tests Results		Surgery

Important observations

Dog Health Record

Breed			Groomer		
Veterinarian		Emergency Veterinary Services			
Date	Physical Test Result	Fecal Test Result	Wormer Given	Heartworms Tests Results	Surgery

Important observations

Dog Health Record

Breed				Groomer		
Veterinarian			Emergency Veterinary Services			
Date	Physical Test Result	Fecal Test Result	Wormer Given	Heartworms Tests Results	Surgery	

Important observations

Dog Health Record

Breed			Groomer		
Veterinarian		Emergency Veterinary Services			
Date	Physical Test Result	Fecal Test Result	Wormer Given	Heartworms Tests Results	Surgery

Important observations

Dog Health Record

Breed			Groomer		
Veterinarian		Emergency Veterinary Services			

Date	Physical Test Result	Fecal Test Result	Wormer Given	Heartworms Tests Results	Surgery

Important observations

Dog Health Record

Breed				Groomer		
Veterinarian			Emergency Veterinary Services			
Date	Physical Test Result	Fecal Test Result	Wormer Given	Heartworms Tests Results	Surgery	

Important observations

Dog Health Record

Breed				Groomer		
Veterinarian			Emergency Veterinary Services			
Date	Physical Test Result	Fecal Test Result	Wormer Given	Heartworms Tests Results	Surgery	

Important observations

Dog Health Record

Breed				Groomer	
Veterinarian		Emergency Veterinary Services			
Date	Physical Test Result	Fecal Test Result	Wormer Given	Heartworms Tests Results	Surgery

Important observations

Dog Health Record

Breed			Groomer		
Veterinarian		Emergency Veterinary Services			
Date	Physical Test Result	Fecal Test Result	Wormer Given	Heartworms Tests Results	Surgery

Important observations

Dog Health Record

Breed			Groomer		
Veterinarian		Emergency Veterinary Services			
Date	Physical Test Result	Fecal Test Result	Wormer Given	Heartworms Tests Results	Surgery

Important observations

Dog Health Record

Breed				Groomer		
Veterinarian		Emergency Veterinary Services				
Date	Physical Test Result	Fecal Test Result	Wormer Given	Heartworms Tests Results	Surgery

Important observations

Dog Health Record

Breed				Groomer		
Veterinarian			Emergency Veterinary Services			
Date	Physical Test Result	Fecal Test Result	Wormer Given	Heartworms Tests Results	Surgery	

Important observations

Dog Health Record

Breed			Groomer		
Veterinarian			Emergency Veterinary Services		
Date	Physical Test Result	Fecal Test Result	Wormer Given	Heartworms Tests Results	Surgery

Important observations

Dog Health Record

Breed				Groomer		
Veterinarian			Emergency Veterinary Services			
Date	Physical Test Result	Fecal Test Result	Wormer Given	Heartworms Tests Results	Surgery	

Important observations

Dog Health Record

Breed			Groomer		
Veterinarian		Emergency Veterinary Services			
Date	Physical Test Result	Fecal Test Result	Wormer Given	Heartworms Tests Results	Surgery

Important observations

Dog Health Record

Breed				Groomer		
Veterinarian			Emergency Veterinary Services			
Date	Physical Test Result	Fecal Test Result	Wormer Given	Heartworms Tests Results	Surgery

Important observations

Dog Health Record

Breed				Groomer	
Veterinarian		Emergency Veterinary Services			
Date	Physical Test Result	Fecal Test Result	Wormer Given	Heartworms Tests Results	Surgery

Important observations

Dog Health Record

Breed				Groomer		
Veterinarian		Emergency Veterinary Services				
Date	Physical Test Result	Fecal Test Result	Wormer Given	Heartworms Tests Results	Surgery	

Important observations

Dog Health Record

Breed			Groomer		
Veterinarian		Emergency Veterinary Services			
Date	Physical Test Result	Fecal Test Result	Wormer Given	Heartworms Tests Results	Surgery

Important observations

Dog Health Record

Breed				Groomer		
Veterinarian			Emergency Veterinary Services			
Date	Physical Test Result	Fecal Test Result	Wormer Given	Heartworms Tests Results	Surgery	

Important observations

Dog Health Record

Breed				Groomer		
Veterinarian		Emergency Veterinary Services				
Date	Physical Test Result	Fecal Test Result	Wormer Given	Heartworms Tests Results	Surgery	

Important observations

Dog Health Record

Breed				Groomer		
Veterinarian			Emergency Veterinary Services			
Date	Physical Test Result	Fecal Test Result	Wormer Given	Heartworms Tests Results	Surgery

Important observations

Dog Health Record

Breed   **Groomer**

Veterinarian   **Emergency Veterinary Services**

Date	Physical Test Result	Fecal Test Result	Wormer Given	Heartworms Tests Results	Surgery

Important observations

Dog Health Record

Breed				Groomer		
Veterinarian			Emergency Veterinary Services			
Date	Physical Test Result	Fecal Test Result	Wormer Given	Heartworms Tests Results	Surgery	

Important observations

Dog Health Record

Breed				Groomer	
Veterinarian			Emergency Veterinary Services		
Date	Physical Test Result	Fecal Test Result	Wormer Given	Heartworms Tests Results	Surgery

Important observations

Dog Health Record

Breed				Groomer		
Veterinarian			Emergency Veterinary Services			
Date	Physical Test Result	Fecal Test Result	Wormer Given	Heartworms Tests Results	Surgery

Important observations

Dog Health Record

Breed				Groomer		
Veterinarian			Emergency Veterinary Services			
Date	Physical Test Result	Fecal Test Result	Wormer Given	Heartworms Tests Results	Surgery	

Important observations

Dog Health Record

Breed			Groomer		
Veterinarian		Emergency Veterinary Services			
Date	Physical Test Result	Fecal Test Result	Wormer Given	Heartworms Tests Results	Surgery

Important observations

Dog Health Record

Breed				Groomer	
Veterinarian			Emergency Veterinary Services		
Date	Physical Test Result	Fecal Test Result	Wormer Given	Heartworms Tests Results	Surgery

Important observations

Dog Health Record

Breed				Groomer		
Veterinarian			Emergency Veterinary Services			
Date	Physical Test Result	Fecal Test Result	Wormer Given	Heartworms Tests Results	Surgery	

Important observations

NOTES